SEPTOPLASTY HEALING FOODS

Complete Guide Unlocking The Secrets Of Nutrition To Rapid Healing After Surgery Success, Nourishing Meal Plans, Recipes, Tips For Optimal Health Wellness

DR. ALLAN FREDA

Contents

Readers can expect to get expert tips on how to make a healthy diet that will help them recover from septoplasty. It has meal plans to make eating easier and more likely to happen, healing recipes that are meant to give you the nutrients you need, and health advice for after you're better.

With its tried-and-true advice and all-around approach, this book is a great resource for people who have just been told they need septoplasty. It gives them the tools they need to make the most of their food after surgery for faster recovery and long-lasting health benefits.

Disclaimer

The information in this book is for informational purposes only and should not replace professional medical advice, diagnosis, or treatment. Always consult your physician or a qualified health provider regarding any medical concerns. Do not disregard professional medical advice or delay seeking it based on information in this book.

The author does not endorse or have affiliations with any mentioned entities. References are for informational purposes only.

Consult your healthcare provider before making dietary or lifestyle changes, especially during recovery from surgery, as individual needs vary.

Results may vary, and the information provided is not guaranteed to produce specific outcomes.

By reading this book, you acknowledge and agree to consult your healthcare provider before implementing any information herein.

For further guidance, consult your healthcare provider or reputable medical websites for reliable information on surgery recovery diets.

CHAPTER 1
WHAT SEPTOPLASTY IS AND HOW IT WORKS

A deviated septum is when the thin wall (nasal septum) between your nose is moved to one side, making it hard to breathe and other problems. Septoplasty is a surgery used to fix this problem. The goal of this treatment is to straighten the septum, which will improve airflow and help with problems like stuffy noses, snoring, and breathing problems. The treatment is usually done with either local or general anesthesia, and each person has a different recovery time.

A Brief Look at Septoplasty

Septoplasty is a common surgery that is suggested for people whose nasal septum is significantly deviated. This can be due to an injury, a birth defect, or a problem with the structure of the nose. It is often done along with other nasal treatments, like turbinate reduction or sinus surgery, to fix other problems with the nose. To get to the septum, the surgeon makes an incision inside the ears.

He or she then cuts away any extra bone or cartilage and straightens the septum as needed.

Once the cuts are healed, the nose packing may be put in to help the septum during the first few weeks of healing.

What to Expect While You Get Better

The time it takes to heal after septoplasty depends on things like how extensive the surgery was, the person's health, and how well they followed the after-surgery care directions. After surgery, patients often have swelling, stuffy noses, and slight pain in the days that follow. If nasal packing is used, it is usually taken out within a few days.

During the first few days of healing, patients may be told to avoid heavy lifting and activities that are too hard on their bodies. Most people can do light activities again in a week, but they should stay away from activities that could hurt their nose for a few weeks. It could take weeks or months to fully recover. During that time, the tissues in the nose slowly heal and breathing gets better.

For people who have had septoplasty or other surgeries, nutrition is very important for their recovery. A healthy, well-balanced diet full of vital nutrients helps tissues heal, lowers inflammation, and strengthens the immune system. This speeds up recovery and lowers the risk of complications. It's also important to stay hydrated to keep your body healing properly and avoid problems like dryness and crusting in the nose passages.

A complete guide to the best diet after surgery for people who have just been diagnosed, with healing recipes, meal plans, and expert advice for long-term health.

Eating a healthy diet can help you heal faster after having a septoplasty and improve your general health.

Here is a complete guide to the best food after surgery, with meal plans, healing recipes, and long-term health tips from experts.

Understanding the Healing Process: It's important to understand the healing process after a septoplasty before getting into specific food suggestions. As soon as surgery is over, the body starts a complicated set of processes to heal harmed tissues, reduce swelling, and protect against possible infections. Good nutrition gives these processes the building blocks they need to work well, which helps with healing and keeps problems to a minimum.

Why Nutrient-Rich Foods Are Important: Nutrient-rich foods are very important for helping the body heal itself. Eating a range of fruits, veggies, lean proteins, whole grains, and healthy fats gives your body the vitamins, minerals, antioxidants, and phytonutrients it needs to repair tissues, lower inflammation, and keep your immune system working well.

Also, getting enough protein is especially important for treating wounds and repairing damaged tissues.

Healing Foods and Recipes: The healing foods listed below can help your body heal even faster after surgery. Citrus fruits, bell peppers, broccoli, and other foods high in vitamin C help the body make collagen and mend tissues.

Omega-3 fatty acids, which can be found in fatty fish, flaxseeds, and walnuts, can help lower pain and swelling by blocking certain enzymes. Adding garlic, ginger, turmeric, and other herbs and spices that are known to reduce inflammation and boost the immune system can also help the body heal and lower its risk of getting illnesses.

Meal Planning for the Best Recovery: Making plans for healthy meals and snacks is important for getting the nutrition you need and helping your body heal after a septoplasty.

At each meal, try to eat a range of healthy foods, such as lean proteins, whole grains, colorful fruits and veggies, and healthy fats. Try out different recipes and ways of cooking to keep meals fun and interesting while still making sure you get enough nutrients.

Tips from Experts for Long-Term Health: Eating well is important for long-term health and good oral health, not just in the days after surgery.

Cutting back on processed foods, sugary snacks, and fats that are bad for you can help lower inflammation and improve your health as a whole. Drink enough water throughout the day to stay hydrated, and think about adding probiotic-rich foods like yogurt, kefir, and fermented veggies to your diet to help your gut stay healthy and your immune system works well.

Finally, putting nutrition first and eating a healthy diet full of healing foods is important for speeding up the healing process after septoplasty. People can improve their general health after surgery, speed up the healing process, and lower their risk of complications by eating nutrient-dense foods, following expert meal plans, and putting long-term wellness strategies into action.

CHAPTER 2
THE BASICS OF HEALING FOODS

A person's healing nutrition is very important for getting better after surgery, especially if they had a treatment like septoplasty to fix problems in their nasal passage. Food is one of the most important things that can help the body heal, reduce inflammation, and boost the immune system. Finding out about the basic ideas behind healing foods, using items that are high in nutrients, and planning a diet around these ideas are all important parts of taking care of yourself after surgery.

How to Use Healing Foods

Healing foods are those that have qualities that can help the body's natural healing processes. These foods usually have a lot of important nutrients, antioxidants, and anti-inflammatory substances that help the body heal tissues, keep the immune system working well, and lower the risk of complications after surgery. It's important to focus on whole, raw foods because they contain many of the vitamins, minerals, and phytonutrients that your body needs to heal. Also, choosing foods that are high in water can help you stay hydrated, improve circulation, and get rid of toxins from your body. It's also important that healing foods are easy to digest, gentle on the stomach, and good for digestive health since digestive problems can make it harder for the body to receive the nutrients that it needs to heal.

Ingredients High in Nutrients

Incorporating a range of nutrient-dense foods into the diet after surgery is very important for helping the body heal. Protein, vitamin C, zinc, vitamin A, and other essential nutrients are very important for wound healing, making collagen, and keeping the immune system healthy. Fruits and vegetables that are high in vitamin C, like bell peppers, oranges, and citrus fruits, help tissues heal and fight oxidative stress. Zinc is an important mineral for building collagen and keeping your immune system healthy. It can be found in large amounts in foods like lean meats, fish, nuts, and seeds.

Vitamin A-rich foods, like carrots, sweet potatoes, and dark leafy greens, help keep the skin and mucous healthy, which is very important for healing after surgery. Also, eating lean protein sources like chicken, fish, tofu, and beans gives you the amino acids your body needs to heal itself and fight off disease.

What You Need to Know About a Healing Diet

After a septoplasty, a healing diet should be based on the basic nutrients that your body needs for full recovery and long-term health. Whole grains like oats, quinoa, and brown rice are great sources of complex carbohydrates that keep you going and give your body the energy it needs to heal. Including a lot of different coloured fruits and veggies also gives you a wide range of vitamins, minerals, and phytonutrients, which help your immune system work better and reduce inflammation. Avocados, nuts, seeds, and olive oil are all good sources of healthy fats that are needed for hormone production, cell membrane stability, and the absorption of fat-soluble vitamins that are important for healing. Also, staying hydrated is important for getting rid of toxins, keeping electrolyte balance, and supporting cell function. This shows how important it is to drink plenty of water and refreshing drinks like herbal teas and broths.

Following the principles of healing nutrition, including nutrient-dense foods, and planning a diet around the building blocks of healing can help people who have had septoplasty recover faster, boost their immune systems, and stay healthy in the long run.

CHAPTER 3
IMPORTANT NUTRIENTS FOR RECOVERY

It's impossible to say enough about how important a well-balanced diet is for care after a septoplasty.

Essential nutrients are very important for helping the body heal after surgery. They help repair tissues, boost the immune system, and speed up the recovery process generally.

Making sure you get enough proteins, vitamins, and minerals is very important to speed up mending and avoid problems. This detailed guide talks about the important nutrients needed for recovery after a septoplasty.

It covers vitamins that help wounds heal, minerals that help tissues repair, and the role of protein in the healing process.

Vitamins are important for the body's wound-healing processes and carry out many functions at different times of the healing process.

There are many vitamins, but some stand out because they help wounds heal very quickly. Vitamin C, for example, is well-known for being an antioxidant and a key part of collagen production, a protein that is needed to heal wounds and grow new tissue. Ensuring you get enough vitamin C after having a septoplasty can help your body fight off infections, speed up wound healing, and improve your general recovery. Vitamin A is also very important for epithelialization, which is the process of growing new tissue over a cut.

Vitamin A helps the healing process after septoplasty by encouraging cell differentiation and growth. This makes it easier for the mucosal tissues to grow back.

Vitamin E is also a powerful antioxidant that helps protect cell membranes from oxidative damage.

This creates an ideal setting for wound healing. Vitamin-rich foods like oranges, fresh greens, carrots, nuts, and seeds can help wounds heal faster and better after a septoplasty.

Minerals to Help Repair Tissue

Minerals are also an important part of nutrition after a septoplasty because they help tissues heal, the immune system work, and the body's general functions. Out of all the minerals, zinc stands out as one of the most important nutrients for wound healing. Zinc is an important cofactor for many enzymes that help make DNA, RNA, and proteins, which are needed for tissue repair and regrowth. Zinc also has immunomodulatory effects that make the body's defences stronger against germs and lower the risk of getting an infection after surgery. Zinc-rich foods, like lean meats, fish, legumes, nuts, and whole grains, can help wounds heal better and speed up the recovery process after a septoplasty. Iron is also very important for moving and using oxygen, which helps tissues get oxygen and speeds up the metabolism of cells, which is necessary for wound healing. Making sure you eat enough iron-rich foods like beans, leafy greens, red meat, chicken, and fortified cereals can help prevent anemia after surgery and help tissues heal properly after a septoplasty.

Protein Is Important for Healing

Proteins are the building blocks of tissues and are essential for the creation, growth, and upkeep of cells. Regarding recovery from a septoplasty, getting enough protein is very important for promoting the best wound healing and tissue regrowth. Protein helps the body heal in many ways. It helps make collagen, keeps the immune system working, and speeds up enzyme processes that are necessary for tissue repair. Protein also helps keep lean muscle mass, which lessens the negative effects of stress and paralysis caused by surgery.

Protein options that are high in quality, like lean meats, poultry, fish, eggs, dairy products, legumes, and tofu, can help people who have had septoplasty meet their higher protein needs during the healing phase. You can also get more protein by adding protein-rich snacks and vitamins to your diet.

This is especially helpful for people who need more protein or who are not hungry after surgery. Prioritizing and increasing protein-rich foods can be very helpful in speeding up wound healing, lowering the risk of complications after surgery, and supporting long-term recovery and health after a septoplasty.

CHAPTER 4
ADDING HERBS AND SPICES FOR HEALTH

When recovering from a septoplasty, adding healing herbs and spices to your diet can help a lot with the healing process and improve your general health. Learning about the healing qualities of different herbs and spices, how to use them in recovery meals, and how to make recipes that feature these ingredients are all important parts of a complete plan for improving your diet after surgery.

How Herbs and Spices Can Help Your Health:

Herbs and spices have been used for hundreds of years to make food taste better and for medical purposes. In the context of recovering from septoplasty, some herbs and spices have healing qualities that can help speed up the process and ease pain.

Turmeric, which is known for being anti-inflammatory and antioxidant, can help lower inflammation after surgery and speed up the healing of tissues. Ginger is another strong ingredient that can help with digestion and reducing inflammation. It can also help with nausea after surgery and make digestion better, which is important for a quick recovery. Herbs like thyme and rosemary also have chemicals that kill microbes, which may lower the risk of getting an infection after surgery. By learning about the specific health benefits of each plant and spice, they can be carefully added to the diet after a septoplasty to help the body heal faster.

Uses in cooking for recovery meals:

Incorporating herbs and spices into recovery meals not only makes them taste better, but they also help the body heal faster. You can easily add these items to a lot of different foods, like salads, smoothies, soups, and stews. You can add fresh herbs like cilantro, basil, and parsley to soups and sauces to make them taste better and give you more vitamins and minerals. Spices like cinnamon and nutmeg can make muesli or yogurt taste better, which can help you feel better and eat better while you're healing. Turmeric can be added to savory dishes like curries or roasted veggies to make them taste better and help your body heal. By adding these foods to their daily meals, people who have had septoplasty can get the most nutrients and help their bodies heal faster.

Recipes that use herbs and spices that are good for you:

Making recipes with healing herbs and spices is a great way to make sure you eat a variety of healthy foods after surgery. Using fresh herbs and spices together can make simple but tasty meals that taste better and help the body heal. For instance, lentil soup with turmeric and ginger in it not only warms you up and makes you feel better, but it also has powerful anti-inflammatory qualities. Garlic, thyme, and rosemary roasted veggies are not only delicious, but they also help the immune system work better and heal wounds faster. Herbal teas with chamomile and peppermint can help with stomach problems and make you feel more relaxed, which is very important for healing. By adding these healing recipes to a patient's post-septoplasty meal plan, doctors can make sure they get all the nutrients and healing benefits they need to get better.

Adding healing herbs and spices to your diet after a septoplasty is a great way to speed up your recovery and improve your health in the long run. Learning about the healing qualities of different herbs and spices, using them in cooking, and making healing recipes are all important parts of a complete approach to nutrition after surgery. By adding these foods to their daily meals, patients can help their bodies heal and improve their quality of life while they are recovering and afterward as well.

CHAPTER 5
HOW TO MAKE NOURISHING SOUPS AND BROTHS

Since a long time ago, people have known that soups and broths can help the body heal, especially after surgery like septoplasty. These liquid-based foods help the healing process in many ways by giving people who are going through the struggles of recovery important nutrients, fluids, and comfort. Figuring out how important it is to eat healthy soups and broths after surgery is important for speeding up recovery and improving general health.

Soups and broths can help you get better:

Soups and broths can help you heal faster after a septoplasty in many ways. For starters, these liquid-based foods are easy to digest, which is important for people who have recently had surgery because their digestive system may be weak for a while. While soups and broths are an easy way to get nutrients, they don't put too much stress on the digestive system. This lets the body focus its energy on healing. Soups and broths are also very high in water, which helps keep you from becoming dehydrated, which can slow down healing and make pain after surgery worse. Staying hydrated is important for keeping your health in general and helping your body heal.

Soups and broths also have a lot of vitamins, minerals, and amino acids, which are all important for healing tissues, keeping your immune system healthy, and making new cells. People who are getting a septoplasty can make sure their bodies get all the nutrients they need to heal faster and better by eating soups and broths that are high in nutrients.

Broth recipes that are high in nutrients:

Making broths that are high in nutrients is an easy and effective way to speed up healing after surgery. There is a famous recipe that calls for cooking bones, like chicken or beef bones, with aromatic vegetables and herbs in water for a long time.

By cooking the bones slowly, collagen, gelatin, and other healthy substances can be extracted, making a broth that is both tasty and full of nutrients. You can also make vegetable-based broths by cooking different veggies in water until they are soft, like celery, onions, garlic, and carrots.

Adding herbs and spices like thyme, rosemary, and turmeric to the soup not only makes it taste better, but it also makes it healthier. Incorporating seaweed like kombu or nori into broth recipes can also give you extra minerals, especially iodine, which is important for your thyroid and general health. Individuals can make their broths with high-quality ingredients, adjusting the recipes to suit their nutritional needs and tastes.

This makes sure that they get the best nutrition needed for healing after surgery.

In addition to broths that are high in nutrients, many other types of comforting soup can help you heal from surgery. Classic choices like veggie soup and chicken noodle soup are not only comforting, but they are also full of nutrients that help the body heal and recover.

Soups like chicken noodle soup are a good source of protein from the chicken, carbs from the noodles, and a variety of vitamins and minerals from veggies like onions, carrots, and celery. Adding things like ginger and garlic to soups can also help reduce inflammation and boost the immune system, which is especially helpful while you're healing. Additionally, creamy soups made from pureed veggies like cauliflower or butternut squash can be soothing and healthy for people with sensitive digestive systems. People who have had septoplasty can find a variety of tasty and healing foods to help them on their way to recovery by trying out different types of soup and playing with the ingredients.

 adding healthy soups and broths to your diet after surgery is an important part of making sure you heal properly and stay healthy in the long run. These liquid-based foods have many benefits, such as being easy to digest, keeping you hydrated, and providing important nutrients that help the body heal itself. By making nutrient-dense broths and trying out different kinds of warming soup, people can make sure they get all the nutrients they need for a quick and easy recovery. People who have had septoplasty can improve their general health and set themselves up for a healthy and happy future by paying attention to their diet and nutrition.

CHAPTER 6
SMOOTHIES AND JUICES THAT HEAL

During recovery from a septoplasty, a surgery used to fix a misaligned septum, it is important to pay close attention to what you eat to help your body heal and stay healthy. repair smoothies and juices can help with recovery and speed up the body's repair processes. These liquid nutrition choices are great for your health because they help with digestion, vitamin absorption, and staying hydrated. They are also a great addition to a diet plan after surgery.

The Power of Liquid Food:

There are many benefits to a liquid diet, especially after surgery when the body may have trouble chewing or digesting solid foods. Smoothies and drinks are great ways to get a lot of vitamins, minerals, antioxidants, and water, all of which are important for healing and keeping the immune system strong. The process of blending or juicing also breaks down the cells of fruits, veggies, and other ingredients, which makes it easier for the body to absorb their nutrients.

This higher bioavailability makes sure that the nutrients are used effectively, which helps with tissue repair and regrowth, which are important parts of the healing process after a septoplasty.

How to Make Healing Smoothies:

To make healing smoothies, you need to carefully choose items that not only taste great but also have health benefits that can help you get better.

Citrus fruits, berries, and leafy greens are all high in vitamins C and E. Eating these foods can help your immune system and lower inflammation, which are both very important for healing after surgery.

Also, adding protein sources like Greek yogurt, nut butter, or plant-based protein shakes to your diet can help your muscles and tissues heal.

Anti-inflammatory ingredients, such as turmeric or ginger, may also be helpful additions.

These can help ease pain after surgery and speed up the mending process. Putting these ingredients together in the right amounts makes smoothies that are both tasty and good for you. The smoothies provide the body with the nutrients it needs to heal itself, and they also look good.

Fresh Juice Mixes to Help You Get Better:

Freshly squeezed drinks are another way to get concentrated nutrition that can help your body heal after a septoplasty.

Fruits and veggies can be juiced to get their powerful vitamins, minerals, and enzymes. The result is a nutrient-dense drink that is easy to digest.

To make juices that will help you recover, you need to focus on using items that are known to be healing and good for you. Eating a range of colorful fruits and veggies will give you a wide range of vitamins, minerals, and antioxidants, all of which are important for keeping your immune system strong and helping tissues heal. For instance, carrots, beets, kale, and pineapple can give you a powerful mix of vitamins A, C, and K, as well as substances that reduce inflammation, such as bromelain and beta-carotene.

Adding plants like parsley or cilantro can also make the juice healthier by adding more nutrients and anti-inflammatory and detoxifying properties.

By trying out different combinations of fresh fruits and vegetables, people can make tasty, nutrient-dense juices that help them recover from surgery and stay healthy in the long run.

 healing smoothies and juices are an easy and effective way to get the nutrients you need to help your health after a septoplasty. People can improve their diet to help tissues heal, lower inflammation, and support general health by using the power of liquid nutrition and adding ingredients that are known to be healing.

Healing smoothies and drinks are great for helping you get better and stay healthy in the long term, whether you eat them as a snack or as part of a full meal plan.

CHAPTER 7
MEALS THAT ARE EASY TO BREAK DOWN

Septoplasty is surgery that straightens out a crooked septum. After surgery, you need to pay close attention to your post-operative care, which includes what you eat. Eating foods that help tissues heal, lower inflammation, and improve digestion can speed up the mending process after septoplasty. This detailed guide goes into detail about the idea of septoplasty healing foods, focusing on simple meals that help with healing and ease pain.

Easy Foods to Digest:

After having septoplasty, it's important to eat meals that are easy for your body to digest so that you don't have to deal with stomach pain and can help it heal faster. By choosing meals that are easy on the stomach, you can help avoid problems after surgery and improve your general health.

Meals that are easy to digest usually include foods that are low in fat, fiber, and spices, all of which can make the digestive system sore. Adding lean proteins, cooked veggies, and whole grains to your diet can help you get the nutrients you need without putting too much stress on your digestive system.

Foods that are easy on stomachs:

For people who have had septoplasty, it is very important to choose soft foods that are easy to digest. These foods usually have mild tastes and textures, which makes them great for people with sensitive stomachs. Simple foods that are gentle are steamed vegetables like zucchini or carrots, lean meats like chicken or fish, and cooked grains like rice or quinoa. Adding fruits that are easy to stomach, like bananas or applesauce, can also help your body absorb vitamins and minerals without making digestive problems worse. Picking foods that are well-cooked and don't have any extra sauces or spices added can help your body heal even more.

Comfort Food Recipes That Are Soft and Pureed:

In the early stages of healing from a septoplasty, soft and pureed recipes can help with comfort and nutrition without putting too much stress on the surgical site.

These recipes are especially helpful for people who may have trouble chewing or eating after surgery because they are sore or swollen. Soups that have been pureed, like veggie bisque or butternut squash soup, are comforting and easy to eat and digest.

In the same way, smoothies made with soft fruits, yogurt, and protein powder can be a healthy meal alternative for people who aren't hungry or have a lot of energy.

Adding soft and pureed foods to the diet after surgery can help the body heal and make sure that it gets enough nutrients while it's healing.

After a septoplasty, people often have digestive problems because of things like anesthesia, painkillers, and changes in the way they eat.

There are, however, several things that can be done to control these symptoms and help digestion while you're healing.

Eating smaller meals more often can make digestion easier, which can help the body absorb nutrients better and get rid of bloating.

Also, staying hydrated by having lots of water or herbal tea can help keep your digestive system healthy and stop you from getting constipated. Staying away from foods that make your stomach hurt, like spicy or fatty foods, can also help ease your symptoms and speed up your healing.

Overall, watching what you eat and doing things to help your digestive system can make the time after surgery better and help you stay healthy in the long run after septoplasty.

 the idea of septoplasty healing foods includes choosing meals that are easy to digest and help with mending while minimizing stomach pain. By eating soft, pureed foods that are good for sensitive stomachs and following tips for dealing with gut pain, people can make the most of their post-surgery diet for long-term health. If you focus on eating mindfully and eating foods that are high in nutrients, they can help you heal and stay healthy while you're recovering from septoplasty.

CHAPTER 8
BREAKFASTS THAT GIVE YOU ENERGY

For healing after a septoplasty, you need more than just medical care. You also need to pay attention to what you eat. A lot of people think of breakfast as the most important meal of the day. It helps your body get going and gives you energy for the day. Those who are recovering from septoplasty need to eat energizing breakfasts even more because they help refill important nutrients, speed up healing, and give people more energy overall.

Ideas for Breakfast Meals in the Morning

For the best nutrition after a septoplasty, your breakfast should include a mix of macronutrients, vitamins, and minerals. Whole grains, lean proteins, healthy fats, and fresh fruits and veggies are all important for helping the body heal. Adding sliced nuts and mixed berries to muesli gives you complex carbohydrates for long-lasting energy, as well as protein and antioxidants that are important for healing tissues. Also, fried eggs with avocado, whole grain toast, and other healthy fats make for a protein-rich meal that also helps the body absorb fat-soluble vitamins.

Recipes for a Healthy Breakfast

It doesn't have to be hard to make healthy breakfast recipes after a septoplasty. Simple foods that are good for you are easy to work into your morning routine. Putting together a shake with Greek yogurt, spinach, banana, and a scoop of protein powder is an easy way to get nutrients without making your stomach hurt. If you want something tasty, a vegetable omelet cooked in olive oil with bell peppers, spinach, and mushrooms is a great way to get the vitamins and minerals your body needs to heal. Adding a side of whole grain toast or a small amount of quinoa to these recipes will help you feel full and pleased by adding fiber and other nutrients.

It's normal to feel tired after having a septoplasty because your body is putting its energy into healing. Adding foods that are known to give you energy can help fight this tiredness and improve your health as a whole. Iron-rich foods, like lean meats, poultry, fish, and leafy veggies, are important for keeping blood oxygen levels healthy and fighting fatigue after surgery.

Breakfasts that are high in complex carbohydrates, like whole grains, sweet potatoes, and beans, can give you energy that lasts all day. Vitamin C-rich foods, like citrus fruits, cherries, and kiwis, also help the body absorb iron and boost the immune system, both of which are important for full healing after a septoplasty.

 energizing breakfasts are very important for healing after a septoplasty because they provide important nutrients, boost energy, and support general health.

 Including breakfast recipes that are balanced and foods that are known to give you energy in the morning is the best way to start getting better and staying healthy in the long run. People who have recently had surgery can improve their quality of life and speed up their healing by focusing on nutrient-dense foods and thoughtful eating.

CHAPTER 9
SNACKS AND SIDES THAT ARE GOOD FOR YOU

Nutrition is one of the most important parts of making sure that you heal properly after a septoplasty. Snacks and side dishes that are high in nutrients are important parts of a well-rounded diet after surgery because they help the body heal.

This complete guide is meant to shed light on healthy snack choices, healing side dishes, and quick and easy recipes that are perfect for people who are always on the go after having a septoplasty.

Snacks that are full of nutrients:

During the delicate phase of recovery after a septoplasty, it's important to feed the body with snacks that are high in nutrients and help the body heal. Snacking on foods that are high in antioxidants, vitamins, and minerals can help reduce inflammation, speed up tissue repair, and boost immune function.

Fresh fruits like kiwis, oranges, and berries are great snacks because they are full of nutrients. For example, kiwis are high in vitamin C, which is an important nutrient that helps make collagen and heal wounds.

 Adding nuts and seeds like flaxseeds, walnuts, and almonds to your diet also gives you protein and omega-3 fatty acids, which are important for healing tissues and keeping your immune system strong.

When paired with sliced cucumbers or carrots, Greek yogurt or cottage cheese is a protein-rich and hydrating snack that can help repair tissues and keep electrolytes in balance. Having hummus with whole grain crackers or vegetable sticks is a great way to get protein, fiber, and anti-inflammatory qualities that will help you recover from surgery.

By adding these healthy snacks to your diet after a septoplasty, you can help your body heal faster and stay healthy overall.

For people recovering from a septoplasty, it is very important to eat nutrient-rich side dishes with their major meals. These side foods not only make meals healthier, but they also help the body heal and stay healthy over time. Leafy greens like spinach, kale, and Swiss chard are great for adding to side salads or sautés because they are full of vitamins A, C, and K, as well as minerals like iron and calcium that are important for healing tissues and keeping the immune system strong. Roasted veggies like broccoli, Brussels sprouts, and sweet potatoes make a hearty and healthy side dish. They are high in antioxidants, fiber, and micronutrients, all of which help the body heal. Whole grains, like quinoa, brown rice, and barley, make healthy side dishes because they contain complex carbohydrates that give you energy and fiber that keeps your digestive system healthy.

Also, adding legumes like black beans, lentils, and chickpeas to side meals not only increases protein intake but also gives you important nutrients like iron, zinc, and folate that you need to recover from surgery. By adding these healing side dishes to your diet after having a septoplasty, you can speed up the healing process and improve your health in the long run.

On-the-go recipes that are quick and easy:

Getting back to normal after a septoplasty can be hard, especially for people who are already very busy. Quick and easy recipes that are designed to help with healing can make meals less stressful while still making sure that essential needs are met. One of these recipes is a smoothie with spinach, banana, Greek yogurt, and almond milk.

This smoothie is full of nutrients like vitamins, minerals, and protein that are important for healing and repairing tissues.

 Overnight oats are a healthy, portable breakfast that can be made with rolled oats, chia seeds, almond milk, and fresh vegetables. They are high in fiber, antioxidants, and omega-3 fatty acids. Making vegetable and quinoa muffins with grated zucchini, carrots, and bell peppers is a quick and easy way to get a variety of nutrients while also making a tasty lunch that you can take with you.

Another quick and easy snack idea is energy balls made from dates, nuts, and seeds. They have the right amount of carbs, protein, and healthy fats to keep you going all day. By adding these quick and easy meals to their diet after having a septoplasty, people can focus on healing while still fitting their busy lives, which will lead to better recovery and better health in the long run.

healthy snacks and side foods are very important for helping the body heal after a septoplasty and for maintaining health over time. By choosing healthy snacks, adding healing side dishes to meals, and making quick and easy recipes for when you're on the go, people can make the most of their diet after surgery to help their recovery and general health.

CHAPTER 10
TASTY MAIN COURSES

Healing foods after a septoplasty are very important for the recovery process because they help the body heal faster and reduce pain. Maintaining a healthy diet is important for your general health, but focusing on certain foods can help you heal faster after septoplasty surgery. Among these, tasty main dishes stand out as an important part of nutrition after surgery because they provide the nutrients, energy, and satisfaction that are needed to help with healing.

Hearty meals to help you get better

Incorporating healthy meals into your diet after septoplasty surgery can help you feel better and speed up the healing process. Choose dishes that are high in lean proteins, whole grains, and colorful veggies to get the nutrients you need and help your body heal.

Soups and stews that are hearty and full of beans, veggies, lean meats, or plant-based proteins can be especially good for you.

These comforting meals are a good source of protein and water, both of which are important for healing and staying healthy after surgery. Additionally, adding herbs and spices to these dishes not only makes them taste better but also has anti-inflammatory qualities that can help reduce swelling and pain after surgery.

Ideas for Meals High in Protein

Protein is important for healing muscles and tissues, so it should be a big part of your meals after a septoplasty. During the recovery time, eating meals that are high in protein can help your body heal and stay healthy overall. Choose lean protein sources like fish, tofu, grilled chicken, or lentils to get the amino acids you need without the extra fat or cholesterol. To make meals that are balanced and healthy, eat these protein sources with whole grains, like quinoa or brown rice, and lots of veggies. Adding dairy or plant-based choices like Greek yogurt, cottage cheese, or almond milk to your diet can also help you get more protein and important vitamins and minerals for healing.

For long-term success with healing foods after a septoplasty, it's important to keep a varied and fun diet. Including recipes that are both tasty and filling in your meal plan can help you stay inspired and make sure you get all the nutrients you need to recover properly. Try using different tasty products and cooking methods to make meals that taste great and help your body heal naturally.

There are a lot of different things you can make, from grilled salmon with a citrus herb marinade to tofu and veggie stir-fry. Adding different textures, colors, and tastes to your meals not only makes them more enjoyable but also makes sure you get a lot of different nutrients that are good for your health and healing.

if you want to heal properly and stay healthy in the long run after a septoplasty, you should focus on eating tasty main courses. By planning your meals around heavy main dishes, protein-packed meals, and tasty recipes, you can make sure your body gets the nutrients it needs to heal while also enjoying meals that are filling and healthy. Remember to talk to your doctor or a registered dietitian about your specific needs and medical background to get personalized nutrition advice.

CHAPTER 11
SWEET TREATS TO HELP YOU GET BETTER

Desserts that are both tasty and good for you:

It's important to eat a balanced diet that helps with recovery and general health while you're healing from septoplasty surgery.

Sweet treats can be a great addition to a diet after surgery, especially if they are full of good things for you. During times of recovery, it can be tempting to reach for sweets.

However, eating desserts that are both satisfying and good for you can help the healing process. Desserts that are high in sugar and fat can provide important nutrients like vitamins, minerals, and antioxidants that help the body heal and fight off disease. People who are getting septoplasty surgery can enjoy sweet treats while also helping their bodies heal by picking desserts that are high in nutrients.

Healthy ways to satisfy your cravings:

People who are having septoplasty surgery may find it hard to meet their sweet tooth cravings without putting their recovery goals at risk. But you can still enjoy desserts without hurting your health if you choose healthy options. When making a healthy dessert, you can often replace unhealthy items with ones that are higher in nutrients, like whole grains, fruits, nuts, and seeds. Not only do these ingredients add flavor and taste, but they also help the body heal by giving it the nutrients it needs and making it feel full. People can satisfy their cravings without feeling guilty if they choose healthy alternatives. This can help them recover from surgery and stay healthy in the long run.

Dessert Recipes That Can Help You Heal:

When planning a diet for after surgery, it's important to include dessert recipes that are good for healing to help with recovery and general health. The items in these recipes should focus on those that are good for you and help your body heal. When choosing healing treat recipes, it's important to include foods that are high in vitamins, minerals, antioxidants, and substances that reduce inflammation. Also, choosing recipes that are easy to swallow and gentle on the stomach can help ease pain after surgery and speed up the healing process. Fruit-based treats, homemade energy bars, yogurt parfaits with nuts and seeds, and whole-grain baked goods are all examples of desserts that can help your body heal. People who have recently had surgery can help their recovery and please their sweet tooth in a healthy way by adding these tasty and healthy desserts to their diet.

CHAPTER 12
HEALTHY EATS AND RECOVERY

It's impossible to say enough about how important careful eating is for recovery after surgery.

After a septoplasty surgery, in which the nasal septum is straightened and repositioned to make breathing easier, the patient's health and healing can be greatly improved by changing the way they eat. Mindful eating means paying full attention to and being present with your body while you eat.

It also means becoming more aware of your hunger cues, taste feelings, and levels of satiety.

Why Mindful Eating Practices Are Important:

People who are recovering from a septoplasty can benefit in many ways from practicing mindful eating. First, it makes you more aware of the foods you eat and how much you eat, which is especially important during the healing phase when your body may have different nutritional needs.

Patients can better control how much food they eat by paying close attention to their hunger and fullness signs. This way, they won't overeat or underheat, which can both slow down the healing process. Mindful eating also encourages people not to judge food, which lets them enjoy and respect every bite without feeling guilty or anxious.

 This helps people in recovery have a healthy relationship with food. Additionally, mindful eating can make meals more enjoyable by focusing on the senses of taste, texture, and smell. This can improve mental health and lower stress levels, both of which are important for the healing process after surgery.

Ways to Enjoy Your Meals While You're Recovering:

By practicing mindful eating, you can greatly improve your dining experience and speed up your healing after septoplasty surgery.

By paying attention to the food's colors, smells, tastes, and textures while you eat, you can help your body feel full. This not only makes meals more enjoyable, but it also helps people be more aware by keeping their attention on the present.

Practicing thanks before meals can also help you feel better and make the whole dining experience better.

Making a conscious effort to be thankful for the healthy food on your plate can help you feel better and connect you more deeply with the healing process.

Another helpful tip is to avoid electronic devices and TV during meals and instead focus on the act of eating and the company of loved ones if you are dining with others.

This makes eating more thoughtful and enjoyable, which helps digestion and nutrient absorption, both of which are important for a full recovery.

Creating a healing environment around food is part of mindful eating habits that can help with recovery after a septoplasty.

This includes many things, like how the food is prepared, how it is presented, and the atmosphere.

All of these things can affect the whole eating experience and help the healing process. When cooking, choosing fresh, nutrient-dense foods can give your body the vitamins, minerals, and enzymes it needs to heal tissues and keep your immune system strong. Incorporating healing foods like fruits, veggies, lean proteins, and whole grains—which are known to reduce inflammation and boost the immune system—can also help the healing process.

Presentation is also an important part of making food a healing setting because meals that look good can make you hungry and improve the dining experience.

Putting time and effort into making food look nice can make eating more enjoyable and encourage people to eat more mindfully.

Creating a calm and peaceful atmosphere during meals with soft lighting, relaxing music, or candles can also help with digestion and relaxation, which can speed up the body's healing process.

By including these things in the dining experience, people can make a safe and caring space that helps them recover from septoplasty surgery and stay healthy in the long run.

CHAPTER 13
MAKING AND PLANNING HEALTHY MEALS

Adopting a diet that helps the body heal and improves general health is an important part of recovering from a septoplasty. Breakfast is one of the most important meals of the day because it starts the metabolism and gives you the nutrients you need for energy and repair. Including a variety of healthy foods can make the healing process go much more smoothly.

Ideas for Breakfast Meals in the Morning

After having a septoplasty, it's important to eat a lot of foods that are high in vitamins, minerals, and fats to help the body heal and fight off illness. Whole grains, like oats or quinoa, can be part of a healthy breakfast because they give you long-lasting energy and fiber, which is important for digestion. Lean proteins, like eggs and Greek yogurt, or plant-based proteins, like tofu and lentils, can help repair and maintain muscles. Adding different fruits and veggies not only makes food taste and feel better but also makes sure that you get a wide range of antioxidants and phytonutrients, which are important for healing and reducing inflammation.

Recipes for a Healthy Breakfast

It doesn't have to be hard to make healthy breakfast recipes after a septoplasty. Overnight oats with fresh berries and nuts on top for extra flavor and texture are a simple and healthy choice. Instead, a hearty omelet with whole-grain toast and lots of vegetables is a filling meal that is high in protein, vitamins, and minerals. If you want to satisfy your sweet tooth, a shake made of leafy greens, fruits, protein powder, and nut butter is an easy and tasty way to get a lot of nutrients.

Foods that give you more energy

Getting enough rest and keeping up your energy levels are very important during the healing phase after septoplasty.

Some things can give you energy all day and help your body heal itself at the same time. Adding complex carbs like whole grains, fruits, and starchy veggies to your diet keeps your glucose levels steady, so you don't lose energy. Iron-rich foods, like lean meats, beans, and leafy greens, also help move oxygen around the body and make energy, which can help with the tiredness that many people feel after surgery. Adding healthy fats from foods like avocados, nuts, and seeds to your meals not only makes them taste better and make you feel fuller, but they also give you a concentrated source of energy.

Making plans for and cooking healing meals

To make sure you follow nutritional rules and easily add healing foods to your diet after a septoplasty, you need to carefully plan and prepare your meals. People can make it easier to feed their bodies while they are recovering by using good meal-planning techniques and stocking a healing kitchen.

How to Plan Meals for Recovery

Planning meals well is very important for making sure you have a steady supply of healthy meals after a septoplasty. Start by making a weekly menu with a range of healthy, nutrient-dense foods that will help you heal and feel better generally. You might want to include foods that are high in zinc, vitamins A and C, and omega-3 fatty acids.

These acids are known to reduce inflammation and boost immune function. Make your meal plans by using online tools or talking to a nutritionist. These plans should be based on your specific dietary needs and tastes.

Batch cooking to save time

Batch cooking is a great way to make meals easier and make sure you have access to healthy foods while you're recovering.

Plan to make a lot of soups, stews, and casseroles with healthy foods every week on a certain day of the week. Make individual servings of these meals and put them in the freezer so they are easy to reheat and eat when required. This method not only saves time and effort, but also cuts down on the use of prepared foods that may slow down the healing process.

What to Put in a Healing Kitchen

Keeping your kitchen stocked with the things you need to make healthy meals is very important after having a septoplasty.

To make sure you always have nutrient-dense foods on hand, stock up on staples like whole grains, lean proteins, fruits, and veggies. Also, keep basic kitchen items like canned tomatoes, beans, and broth on hand so that putting together meals is quick and easy. Buy good cooking appliances and tools, like a blender or food processor, to make it easier to make smoothies and recipes that are good for you.

By preparing a healing kitchen ahead of time, people can easily add healthy foods to their diet after surgery, which helps them recover quickly and stay healthy in the long run.

CHAPTER 14
HELPING WITH LONG-TERM WELLNESS

Following a septoplasty surgery to fix a deviated septum, it is very important to follow a special diet to stay healthy in the long run. Making the change from the diet you were on before surgery to one that helps you heal and helps you recover as much as possible needs careful thought and planning. It is very important to eat foods that help reduce inflammation, boost the immune system, and help tissues heal. As your healthcare provider tells you, you should slowly start eating solid foods again as you move on to a post-recovery diet. You should also make choices that will help your healing and general health.

As the nasal tubes heal after septoplasty, they go through a lot of changes.

Start with foods that are easy to digest, like soups, broths, and pureed veggies, to help this process along. These foods are easy on the digestive system and give you the nutrients you need without making you feel bad. Eating foods that are high in zinc, vitamins A and C, and protein can also help tissues heal and lower the risk of illness. As the body heals and your comfort level allows, slowly add harder foods back into your diet while still focusing on foods that help the body heal.

For long-term health and fitness, it's important to keep up healthy eating habits after having a septoplasty. After the initial time of healing, it's important to focus on a healthy, well-balanced diet that includes a variety of nutrient-dense foods.

To have sustainable eating habits, you need to choose whole, raw foods over processed and sugary foods as much as possible. Adding a variety of fruits, vegetables, whole grains, lean meats, and healthy fats to your diet can help you get all the nutrients you need and stay healthy.

For long-term health, try to eat a lot of antioxidants, vitamins, and minerals. These can help lower inflammation, boost the immune system, and speed up the healing of tissues. To support the body's natural healing processes, stress how important it is to stay hydrated by drinking enough water throughout the day. Also, eat mindfully by doing things like taking your time, chewing your food well, and paying attention to your body's signals for when it's hungry or full. Your body will continue to heal and your health and well-being will improve over time if you change the way you eat.

Recipes for Long-Term Nutrition

Including healing foods in your diet after septoplasty can help you stay healthy and heal as quickly as possible. These recipes focus on using foods that are high in nutrients and help the body heal, reduce inflammation, and stay healthy generally.

Many tasty and healthy meals can help you get better, from warming soups and stews to shakes and salads that are full of nutrients.

A vegetable and lentil soup is a healing food that you might want to try. It is full of vitamins, minerals, and fiber, which are all good for your digestive health and help you heal. In olive oil, sauté garlic, onions, carrots, celery, and celery.

Then, add veggie broth, lentils, and any herbs and spices you like. Let it cook on low heat until the lentils are soft. Then serve it hot for a healthy and satisfying meal. A green smoothie is another choice. It has fruits, leafy veggies, and protein-rich foods like Greek yogurt or tofu. Pour water or almond milk into a blender and add spinach, kale, banana, berries, and your protein of choice. This will make a cool and healthy drink.

In addition to healing foods, meal plans can help you make sure you're eating a healthy, well-balanced diet that helps you heal the best way possible.

You should work with a dietitian or nutritionist to make a meal plan that fits your tastes and wants and gives your body the nutrients it needs to heal.

By adding healing recipes and meal plans to your diet after septoplasty, you can help your body heal better and stay healthy in the long run.

CONCLUSION

When you're recovering from surgery, especially a procedure like septoplasty, you need to take a more comprehensive approach that includes not only medical care but also care for your nutrition and general health. In this detailed guide, we've gone into great detail about how to diet after surgery, giving you information, meal plans, and expert advice that will help you heal and be healthy in the long run.

By learning about the basics of septoplasty and the healing process, as well as the basics of a healing diet, we've shown how important it is to get the right food to help with recovery.

We've talked in detail about healing smoothies and juices, nourishing soups and broths, essential nutrients, and easy-to-digest meals. This way, there are a lot of choices for people with different dietary needs and tastes during the recovery phase.

There is also a connection between mental health and physical recovery, which is why we've stressed the importance of mindful eating and making food a healing setting. It has also been talked about how to plan and make healing meals, support long-term wellness, and switch to a diet after recovery.

This advises beyond the immediate healing period to encourage long-term health and vitality.

When people start their journey after surgery, armed with the information in this guide, they can make choices that will help them recover faster and set them up for a healthy, thriving future.

By following the ideas in this article, people can start on a path of holistic healing that will nourish not only their bodies but also their emotions as they move toward long-term health.